CANCER PREVENTION

Manual with Updated Medical Information

First Edition

Author: Luis Mendoza, MD, PhD

Education is the main pillar in a development that brings significant benefits to people's quality of life. This publication on the prevention of cancer is part of an education program aimed at the general public, cancer patients and health professionals that wish to be better informed on the subject. The goal of this manual is to share the basic concepts relating to cancer and its prevention. The information compiled in this manual is based on scientifically validated data obtained from clinical studies. Thanks to these findings, groups of experts have been able to develop recommendations on the best preventive methods for the different kinds of cancer. These recommendations are collected in this manual.

There is no doubt that the prevention of diseases is an effective way to practice medicine on a large scale. Hence, a good understanding of the risk factors that can cause cancer and knowledge of how to prevent its onset will not only reduce the physical load, the suffering of patients and their families and costs to the cancer patient, but will also lend support to the health system by reducing costs associated with the high mortality and morbidity rates that are currently seen in relation to cancer.

A further objective of this educational manual is to improve the communication between doctors and patients. Better-informed patients are able to voice their questions and concerns better, and in this way they will have greater control over the disease.

This manual will be periodically revised and updated in order to deliver accurate and scientifically validated information. I hope that this manual achieves its objectives and that by educating, it may help combat the terrible cancer scourge that continues to afflict humankind.

TABLE OF CONTENTS

1 What Is Cancer?

Cancer is an unregulated proliferation of cells due to loss of normal controls, resulting in unregulated growth, lack of differentiation, local tissue invasion, and, often, metastasis. - The Merck Manual

Hippocrates, known today as the father of medicine, proposed the humoral theory of medicine. **According to his theory** the body is composed of four fluids: blood, phlegm, yellow bile and black bile. Any imbalance among these fluids was thought to cause disease. Hippocrates attributed cancer to an excess of black bile. He was also the first to use the terms "carcinos" and "carcinoma" to describe tumors, and that is how the term "cancer" came to be used to refer to this particular disease. **The word cancer is derived from the Greek "karkinos" which means** *crab*. Looking into the past, there are signs of cancer that have been found in the bones of mummies from ancient Egypt and Peru, dating back to 3000 BC

It is very common for the general public to confuse the definitions of tumor, cancer, neoplasia, etc. When doctors refer to cancer, neoplasia or malignant tumor, they are talking about the same thing, that is, that the patient has a cancer. When doctors refer to a tumor, they are talking about a patient having some tissue that is showing an abnormal growth. The tumor can be benign or malignant. Benign tumors are normally localized tumors that rarely grow further. On the other hand, a malignant tumor is synonymous with cancer.

2 Types of cancer

More than 200 different types of cancer can be determined by their histology, that is, the study of tissues under the microscope. The medical community together with the World Health Organization has been working for decades toward establishing a histological classification of tumors. Currently, the International Classification of Diseases for Oncology, 3rd Edition, is available for English speaking medical personnel, as well as the Spanish Version (Clasificación Internacional de Enfermedades para Oncología) for Spanish-speaking medical personnel.

More information on the WHO's classification can be found by going to

http://www.who.int/classifications/icd/adaptations/oncology/en/index.html

In general, cancers can be classified into two large categories: solid malignant tumors and hematological (or liquid) tumors.

Most cancers take the name of the organ or cells in which they originate. For example:

Among the hematological malignant tumors, there are cancers of the white blood cells (other than the lymphocytes), which are called leukemias, and cancers of the lymphocytes, which are lymphomas and myeloma.

Among solid tumors, for example, cancer originating in the lungs is called lung cancer. The cancer that originates in the melanocytes (cells that produce a pigment, melanin, found in skin, eyes and hair and whose main function is to block ultraviolet rays) is called melanoma.

Keep in mind that each group of cancers originating in solid or hematological tissue has further subclassifications according to the type of characteristic cell (histology) of which the tumor is formed. An example of this is lung cancer. Lung cancer can be classified into two groups according to its histology (small cell carcinoma and large cell carcinoma), and these can, in turn, be classified into various cancer subtypes.

When we refer to a specific cancer (for example ovarian cancer or renal cancer), we should always remember that there can be different types and that they differ based on their histology, i.e., the study of the tissue under the microscope. Knowing the histological classification of a cancer is vital nowadays in order to establish prognoses and treatments based on the specific type of tumor. Sometimes there are cancers that are difficult to confirm under the microscope, and so it becomes necessary to resort to special immunohistochemical tests: a study of the expression of markers, a study of the chromosomal abnormalities of the tumorous cells etc. and, eventually, a review of the samples, conducted by another more-experienced pathologist.

At this point, we need to highlight the fact that benign tumors never turn into malignant tumors. That is, if a tumor is diagnosed as cancerous, it is because the original cells were malignant. In other words, a malignant tumor, or cancer, always stems from an initial malignant clone. A characteristic of malignant tumors, rather than of benign ones, is that they spread to other parts of the body. These disseminations are called metastases. Tumors that cause metastases are called malignant primary tumors.

3 Naming Tumors

Understanding how doctors name tumors can be difficult. There are certain general rules that are applicable to most tumors. When we refer to a benign tumor, its name always ends with the suffix -oma. It is important not to be confused by the suffix when we talk about sarcomas or blastomas or when the tumor is called carcinoma, as these refer to malignant tumors. Pause for a moment to review Table 1 in order to identify the names of benign and malignant tumors, based on the suffix of a tumor originating from the same tissue.

Table 1

Tissue of Origin	Benign Tumor	Malignant Tumor
skin or mucous membrane	papiloma	squamous-cell carcinoma
glandular epithelium	adenoma	adenocarcinoma
fibrous tissue	fibroma	fibrosarcoma, fibroblastoma
cartilage	chondroma	chondrosarcoma, chondroblastoma
smooth muscle	leiomyoma	leiomyosarcoma, leiomyoblastoma
striated muscle	rhabdomyoma	rhabdomyosarcoma, rhabdomyoblastoma
bone tissue	osteoma	osteosarcoma, osteoblastoma

Aside from the suffixes that help to quickly recognize if the tumor is benign or malignant, doctors also use prefixes. In general, the names for the tumors are created using different prefixes (of Latin origin) that correspond to the tissue or organ where the cancer began its uncontrolled growth (Table 2). For example, the prefix "chondro" means cartilage, so a cancer originating in the cartilage is known as a chondrosarcoma. Similarly, the prefix "adeno" means gland, so a cancer of the glandular cells is known as adenocarcinoma—for example, a breast adenocarcinoma or breast cancer.

Table 2

Prefix	Meaning
adeno-	gland
chondro-	cartilage
erythro-	red blood cells
hemangio-	blood vessels
hepato-	liver
lipo-	fat
lympho-	lymphocytes
melano-	melanocytes
myelo-	bone marrow
myo-	muscle
osteo-	bone

Unfortunately, this rule for naming tumors does not apply to all of them. There are some tumors that are named after the person who discovered them, such as Hodgkin's disease, Wilms' tumor or Ewing's sarcoma. There are other tumors that are named after the cell where they originate, as in the case of tumors of the nervous system: oligodendrogliomas, ependymomas, astrocytomas, etc. These, also, are not named according to the rule that was previously mentioned.

4 Properties of Cancerous Cells

In spite of its diversity, cancer shares a few fundamental properties. Some cancers display each of these properties to different extents. Some others exhibit those properties as the cancer progresses. The common properties of cancers are detailed in the following table.

Table 3

Properties of Cancerous Cells	
Increased and autonomous cellular proliferation	Uncontrolled hyperproliferation of cancerous cells
Insufficient Apoptosis	Apoptosis, or "cellular suicide," is the mechanism by which old or damaged cells normally self-destruct. In cancer, this mechanism is interrupted.
Altered Cellular Differentiation	There are cancers that may also release proteins that under normal conditions are not released; such is the case of the carcinoembryonic antigen seen in colon cancer or the alpha-fetoprotein in liver cancer.
Altered Metabolism	Malignant cells require a lot of resources in terms of energy and nutrients for their exaggerated growth. Carcinogenic cells have an exaggerated increase in the DNA synthesis necessary for cell division and an exaggerated demand of lipids from fatty acids and proteins for the formation

	of new cancerous cells.
Genetic Instability	All types of chromosome malformations, such as deletion, translocation or duplication, are common in cancerous cells.
Immortalization	Cancerous cells can be immortal, that is, they can reach an infinite number of cellular divisions.
Invasion of Other Surrounding Tissue	One of the characteristics of malignant tumors is that they usually invade adjacent structures.
Metastasis in Local Lymph Nodes and Distant Organs	The nutrients and oxygen supply from existing blood vessels are insufficient for tumoral growth. For this reason, cancers trigger neoangiogenesis, which is the growth of new blood vessels. During metastasis, the cancerous cells break away from the primary tumor (lose their contact inhibition and polarization) and migrate through the blood vessels or lymph to distant organs to form new tumors.

5 Risk Factors Related to Cancer

Anything that increases the probability of contracting a disease is called a risk factor. Having a risk factor does not mean that you are going to contract cancer. Not having a risk factor does not mean that you are not going to contract cancer. People who think that they could be at risk should consult their doctor about this.

The risk factors that have been linked to cancer are: endogenous factors, exogenous factors and carcinogenic agents

5.1 Endogenous Factors

Type: The frequency with which different cancers are found present varies depending upon the type. It is estimated that 20% of humans, chickens and laboratory mice have cancer present at some point in their lives, while with pigs, cows and goats the percentage does not exceed 0.5%. The frequency of mammary gland neoplasms in dogs and cats is very high in comparison with other domestic species.

Gender: Being a woman is the greatest risk factor. Women have a more developed mammary gland than men, but what is important is that the cells of this gland are subject to constant stimulation due to factors such as hormonal growth, estrogen and progesterone. Men can have breast cancer but the incidence rate is very low: 100 times less than in women. Thyroid and gallbladder cancers are more common in women than in men.

Age: Certain types of leukemias and tumors in the nervous system are more common in children. Hodgkin's Lymphoma and osteosarcoma are more common in young people. Carcinomas and chronic lymphocytic leukemia are more common in elderly people. The risk of suffering from cancer rises with age. About 18% of breast cancers are diagnosed in people in their 40s and 77% in people over the age of 50. After the age of 75, the risk declines.

Race: Caucasian women have a higher risk of suffering from breast cancer. Blacks and Asians have a lower risk. The real reasons behind this are still unknown. At this point in time lifestyle is thought to be the most influential factor. Prostate cancer is more common in black men than in Caucasian men (the reason is not yet known). A diet that is high in fat content can have an influence in contracting prostate cancer.

Immunological Factors: People with weakened immune systems are more likely to suffer from certain types of cancer. This group includes people who:

- Have had organ transplants and take medications to suppress their immune system in order to prevent the rejection of organs. These patients are prone to developing lymphomas.

- Suffer from HIV or AIDS. In these patients it is common to find Kaposi's sarcoma and other cancers.

- Are born with uncommon medical syndromes that affect their immunity.

Family History: The tendency to develop a tumor in numerous neoplasms such as retinoblastoma, Wilms tumor, breast cancer familiar neurofibromatosis, adenomatous polyposis etc. is inherited.

Recent studies show that about 5 to 10% of breast cancers are hereditary as a result of an alteration in the genes (mutations). The most well-known are: BRCA 1 and BRCA 2. Women who have mutations in these genes have an 80% chance of developing breast cancer during their life, even at a young age. Women with cancer in one breast have a 3 to 4 times greater risk of contracting this disease in the other breast.

Chromosomal Alterations: Chromosomal anomalies without a hereditary tendency imply a greater susceptibility to developing a neoplasm in the diseased. For example: in Down 's syndrome (Trisomy 21) the risk of acute lymphoblastic and myeloblastic leukemia is 15 times greater.

5.2 Exogenous Factors

Environmental Factors: Exposure to ionizing radiation is related to a greater incidence of breast cancer, especially if this occurs before the age of 40. Those between the ages of 10 and 14 are the most susceptible to an increased risk of breast cancer due to ionizing radiation.

The most damaging ionizing radiations are due to:

- Nuclear accidents.

- Radiation therapy treatments in the breast area.

Hormones: The administration of hormonal substitutive therapy to treat the symptoms of menopause is clearly not advised. An increase in the risk of breast cancer has been shown, estimated at 3 additional annual cases per every 1,000 women, or an individual risk increase of 0.3%. This increase in the risk of developing cancer is mostly related to the hormonal substitutive therapy that combines estrogen and progesterone and when this treatment is received over a long period of time (more than 15 years). The risk can increase up to 83%. For this reason, it is currently recommended to avoid the use of hormonal substitutive therapy to fight the symptoms of menopause. Hormonal substitutive therapy can only be considered in low doses and for as short a period of time as possible for women with no family history of breast cancer and with severe menopausal symptoms.

Carcinogenic Agents: Of the 7 million known chemical compounds, 2 million have shown some kind of carcinogenic activity. Moreover, aside from its composition, a substance's ability to produce cancer depends on the dose received and on the duration of exposure to it. Asbestos, arsenic, benezene, cadmium, mercury, nickel, lead, chlorine hydrocarbons, naphthylamine and others (Table 4) are some of the agents with the most common carcinogenic activity. The tar from coal and its derivatives is considered highly carcinogenic. Its steam in some industries (refineries) is associated with a raised incidence of lung cancer among workers. Nowadays it is known that benzopyrene, a chemical substance found in coal, can cause skin cancer in people whose work involves burning coal. Arsenic is associated with lung cancer, therefore workers in copper and cobalt mines, foundries and insecticide factories present a higher than normal incidence of this type of cancer. With workers in industries related to asbestos, the incidence is up to 10 times more than normal.

A substance produced by the fungus Aspergillus flavus, known as aflatoxin, is known to contaminate poorly preserved food and cause liver cancer in some animals. It has been found that in countries where food contamination by mold is common, the incidence of liver and stomach cancer is high.

Cigarettes are the greatest carcinogenic agent in daily life. It has been calculated that lung cancer related death is 6 times more likely to occur in smokers than in non-smokers. Cigarettes are very damaging due to the substances that they contain; nicotine, carbonic acids and oxides and tar. Moreover, they can cause other cancers such as mouth, tongue, esophagus and bladder cancer. The risk of suffering from a cancer due to cigarette consumption generally remains for at least 10 years after having stopped smoking, and in some cases the risk remains for life. 90% of lung cancer deaths are due to this habit. At the same time, second-hand smokers have a greater risk of tumors than the general population.

Alcohol is also considered a carcinogenic agent. Those who drink in excess are at a greater risk of suffering from mouth, esophagus, tongue and liver cancer.

The following table details types and examples of the agents or carcinogens that are known to be able to develop a cancer.

Table 4

Types of Carcinogenic Agents	Examples
Chemical carcinogens	Nickel, cadmium, asbestos, arsenic, mercury, lead, nitrosamines, trichloroethylene, arylamines, benzopyrenes, aflatoxins, reactive oxygen species
Physical carcinogens	Radiation ultraviolet (especially UVB), ionizing radiation
Biological carcinogens	Human papilloma virus, Epstein Bar Virus, Hepatitis B and C, helicobacter pylori and schistosoma mansoni.

Endogenous processes	Oxidation by reactive oxygen species, reduction with antioxidants, reaction with free radicals and inhibition of the repair of oxidation in the DNA, chronic inflation.

Patients who have survived cancer once are susceptible to getting cancer again. The percentage of having a second cancer is 8%. The likely cause of this second cancer risk factor is due to the genetic damage suffered in the cells after chemo and radiotherapy treatments.

6 Risk Factors Whose Correlation to Cancer Development Has Not Been Confirmed

There is currently no conclusive data regarding the relationship between breast cancer incidences and various aspects of daily life such as environmental pollution, smoking, the consumption of some products such as coffee, phytoestrogens or anti-inflammatories, the use of antiperspirant deodorants or the insertion of breast implants.

Caffeine: No study has shown a clear relationship between its consumption and the risk of breast cancer.

Environmental Pollution: There are no conclusive studies on this topic either.

Antiperspirant Deodorants: Currently no scientific study has shown that breast cancer is related to the daily use of antiperspirant deodorants.

Breast Implants: No evidence suggests that there is an increased risk of suffering breast cancer. However, it is important to bear in mind that breast implants make it very difficult to study the mammary tissue in a mammogram.

Infertility Treatment: No effect in the risk of developing breast cancer has been shown. Very recent large studies have confirmed this.

Prolonged Consumption of Anti-inflammatories: No risk relationship between the consumption of anti-inflammatories and the development of cancer has been shown. On the contrary, it seems that they play a part in protecting the body against colon cancer.

Phytoestrogens: The incidence of breast cancer is the lowest in Asian countries such as China or Japan. This is attributed to the high consumption of soy from infancy, which contains weak estrogens. However, there are no conclusive studies on the probable protective effects of these substances. There is no evidence that the consumption of soy or soy products increases the incidence or risk of breast cancer.

Contraceptive Pills: Various studies suggest that the use of contraceptive pills slightly increases the risk of breast cancer, especially in young women. However, the risk disappears after 10 or more years of discontinuing its use. The new contraceptive pills may present a lower risk than the earlier formulations.

Blows to the Breasts No relationship between a trauma to the breast and subsequent breast cancer development is known. A strong blow can produce a hematoma that is later reabsorbed but leaves scar tissue on the skin. It is possible that mammograms will be able to observe this lesion in the future and make room for doubts regarding its nature.

Bra Underwires: No relationship between the use of underwire bras and breast cancer has been shown.

Repeated Mammograms: In order to carry out a mammogram, a small amount of X rays is used. Conducted in such a way, the risk of mammograms causing any damage is low or nonexistent. In general, the benefits of having regular mammograms outweigh the risks.

<u>Underarm Hair Removal:</u> (of any type, principally laser removal): There is no evidence that there could be any relationship between hair removal and breast cancer.

<u>Different Sized Breasts</u>: There is no evidence that any relationship could exist. Having one breast slightly larger than the other is common in women.

<u>Breast Size:</u> There is no evidence that there could be any relationship between breast size and developing breast cancer.

<u>Cell Phones:</u> There is no evidence that any relationship could exist.

7 What is Prevention?

Prevention is defined as the combination of actions aimed at preventing the illnesses from appearing or reoccurring. In fact, it has been shown that some types of cancer can be prevented from developing and can be stopped in the early stages of development. A great deal of suffering and death due to cancer could be prevented with more systematic efforts to reduce the consumption of tobacco, improve diet and physical activity, reduce obesity and increase the use of screening. The American Cancer Association (ACS) estimates that around 170,000 deaths from cancer are caused

by tobacco alone.

8 Data on the Incident Rates of Cancer

Cancer is the main cause of death on a global scale and is a health problem of the first order. In adults, it is the second largest cause of death after cardiovascular diseases and the second among children after accidents. 7.6 million deaths (approximately 13% of the total) are attributed to cancer worldwide. More than 70% of deaths by cancer occurred in low and middle income countries. It is predicted that the number of deaths by cancer will continue to grow worldwide and will exceed 13.1 million in 2030 mainly due to the ageing population.

The main types of most common cancers and those that cause the most deaths worldwide are the following:

- Lung cancer (1.37 million deaths);

- Gastric cancer (736,000 deaths);

- Liver cancer (695,000 deaths);

- Colon cancer (608,000 deaths);

- Breast cancer (458,000 deaths);

- Cervical cancer (275,000 deaths).

9 Most Common Cancers Based on Sex and Age

The most common types of cancer are different for men and women. In both sexes breast, prostate, colon and lung cancer are the most common.

Breast cancer is the most common form of cancer for women and is the cause of 17% of cancer deaths in this type. This is followed by colon, lung, uterine, and ovarian cancer and non-Hodgkin lymphoma in that order. It should be noted here that the incidence of colon cancer in women is lower than in men.

Prostate cancer is the most common cancer in men, however lung cancer is the main cause of cancer related death. This is followed by lung, colon and bladder cancer as well as non-Hodgkin lymphoma and melanoma in that order.

The incidence of cancer in children and adolescents has been increasing for many years. Leukemias, especially of the lymphoid type, malignant tumors in the brain and central nervous system, lymphomas, sarcomas in the soft tissue, and bone tumors (especially bone sarcoma) are the main cancers that develop in children and adolescents.

10 The Importance of Cancer Prevention

The majority of cancers caused by tobacco and alcohol abuse can be completely prevented. Many of the cancers caused by external factors, such as infectious organisms, can also be prevented. A large proportion of colon cancers can be prevented from developing by avoiding the risk factors such as physical inactivity, obesity and the consumption of red and processed meats, along with early detection and the removal of cancerous lesions. The majority of cancers of the uterine canal (cervix) can be prevented with vaccinations against human papillomavirus and also through early detection and the elimination of abnormalities in the uterine canal.

It should be taken into account that 30% of cancer related deaths are due to five risk factors that are behavioral and dietetic: high BMI, reduced intake of fruits and vegetables, lack of physical activity, consumption of tobacco and alcohol.

The consumption of tobacco is the greatest risk factor, and it is the cause of 22% of cancer related deaths worldwide in general, and 71% of worldwide lung cancer related deaths.

Cancers caused by viral infections, such as infections from Hepatitis B (HBV) and C (HCV) or from the human papillomavirus (HPV) are responsible for up to 20% of cancer related deaths in low and middle income countries.

As stated earlier, cancer is one of the main causes of death for humans today. Cancer in its early stages, when it is potentially curable, does not show symptoms and grows in the human body in silence. This is a characteristic of cancer that makes it a terribly dangerous and deadly disease. Even more so when the malignant tumor is quite developed and has spread to other organs, and there still may be no sign of symptoms. A basic medical criterion is that if the tumor is intercepted in its' early stages of development it will not spread, the probability of being cured increases and aggressive oncological treatments with chemotherapy and radiotherapy are avoided. This in turn reduces the costs for the patient and for the health care systems in all countries.

Remember that cancer develops over the years and is not fatal as long as it does not reach advanced stages.

11 Primary Prevention

We can say that there are 2 types of prevention applicable to cancer: primary and secondary prevention. Primary prevention aims to reduce the incidence of cancer by impeding or limiting an individual's exposure to risk factors, or by building up a resistance to them. This objective is mainly achieved using educational strategies that inform people on how to modify risky habits. Primary prevention aims to reduce the incidence of cancer from an epidemiological perspective. This simply means reducing the number of new cases, and avoiding or at least reducing the impact of carcinogenic agents. Along these lines, environmental factors as well as lifestyle habits, such as tobacco use or diet related factors are the aim of primary prevention strategies. In this group there is a new strategy that has attracted a lot of interest over the last few years. This is the strategy known as chemoprevention.

11.1 The Importance of Quitting Smoking

Since 1912 tobacco has been known to be related to lung cancer, a fact supported by solid epidemiological evidence since the 50s. The use of advertisements on cigarette packages dates back to 1965 and the prohibition of advertising on cigarettes dates back to 1970.

These acts along with public health campaigns have had a significant impact in constantly reducing the amount of smokers, by as much as a half since 1950 in the USA. It takes time for the damaging effects of the thousands of carcinogenic chemicals from tobacco to disperse and it was not until 1990 that the incidence of lung cancer in men started to fall.

On a global level, tobacco consumption causes more than 5 million deaths per year, and the current trends show that the consumption of tobacco will cause more than 8 million deaths per year in 2030.

Approximately 20% of the population in the USA is comprised of smokers. Among this group, Native Americans and/or Alaskan natives have the highest percentage of smokers (23%) and Asians are among those who smoke the least. Education plays a part and those with a university level of education smoke less (6%) than those with only a basic level of education (25%). Smoking causes cancer, heart diseases, brain damage and lung diseases (including emphysema, bronchitis and chronic obstruction of the respiratory canals).

Stopping smoking can highly reduce the risk of death by lung cancer, and can also reduce the risk of throat, mouth and especially bladder tumors. Tobacco use is a habit of more than 90% of people with lung cancer, and to treat it, cancer prevention would be the main form of intervention. After 10 years of having broken the habit 30-50% reductions in the risk of suffering from lung cancer can be seen.

Smoking is an addiction. It is easier for light smokers, those who are less addicted, to break the habit. Experts believe that heavy smokers generally need an intense detoxification program that includes counselling, behavioural strategies and therapy with medications such as nicotine and antidepressant substitutions (bupropion).

Much of the information in the public domain is focused on the risks of smoking. Cigar smokers, who do not inhale the tobacco smoke, risk developing the same health problems associated with cigarettes, especially the risks of developing cancers in the mouth or throat. Those who chew tobacco are at risk of developing cancer in the lips and mouth due to the direct contact of carcinogens with the mucosa there. Esophageal cancer is linked to the tobacco carcinogens that dissolve in the saliva, which are swallowed and later come in contact with the esophagus thus starting the development of cancer in this organ.

In the USA different programs have been established to control tobacco use. The main objectives of the campaigns are directed towards:

- Preventing the initial use of tobacco among young people.

- Promoting the necessity of giving up the habit of tobacco use among young people and adults.

- Eliminating the exposure of non-smokers to smokers.

- Identifying and eliminating disproportions in the use of tobacco and in its effects among different groups of the population

Passive exposure to tobacco smoke is also a risk factor for lung cancer. Exposure to second-hand smoke is caused by the smoke coming from a lit cigarette or another tobacco product or the smoke exhaled by smokers. People inhaling tobacco smoke in the environment are exposed to the same cancer producing agents as smokers, although in lower quantities. The inhalation of tobacco smoke in the environment is called involuntary or second-hand smoking. Recent studies demonstrate that in one hour a person can inhale a quantity equivalent to 2 or 3 cigarettes. But young people who can spend many hours enclosed in places where there is excessive smoking are at the greatest risk, given that anyone who is shut up in a place with a lot of smoke such as a bar, nightclub or in a party experiences the equivalent smoking of an entire pack of cigarettes. A second-hand smoker has a 20 to 30 percent greater risk of suffering from lung cancer. This is the reason why health authorities restrict smoking in public spaces.

11.2 The Importance of Changing Eating Habits to Help Prevent Cancer

Breast, colon, endometrial and prostate cancer rates are higher in western countries than in the east. Immigrants from eastern countries and their descendants who acquire American eating habits are at a greater risk of suffering cancer after some time living in the USA. These observations are bases for believing that a change in the diet can, by itself, reduce the incidence of these tumors. Diets that are low in fats, and red meats and high in fruits and vegetables, grant protection due to the protective substances (anticarcinogens) found in vegetables, fruits, nuts and grains. The anticarcinogens found in this type of diet are phenols, components of sulfur and flavones.

The cancer preventing benefits of these diets are theoretical and not yet scientifically confirmed. The latest results in clinical studies indicate that there is no benefit to fiber rich diets and no evidence that a low fat diet can prevent colon and breast cancer respectively. Nor is there any evidence that vitamins, minerals and nutritional supplements in large quantities greater than those in a correct diet have a protective effect. Given that obesity also increases the risk of suffering diabetes, hypertension, heart diseases and premature death, maintaining a healthy weight and increasing physical activity are considered an important strategies for reducing the risk of many chronic diseases, and despite not having a firm basis, it is also recommended as a way of preventing cancer.

11.2.1 Recommended Changes in Eating Habits

In the first place, one should learn to consume food and drink in the right quantities to help reach and maintain a healthy weight. To do this you should familiarize yourself with the standard food portion sizes and read the food product specifications in order to know how many servings can be served.

Only eat small portions of high calorie foods. Be careful with products that are low fat or fat free, as this does not mean low in calories.

Substitute high calorie foods such as hamburgers, pizza, ice cream and sugary drinks with vegetables, fruits and other low calorie foods. Eat 5 or more small portions of vegetables and fruits every day.

Choose grain based foods such as rice, wholegrain bread, pasta and cereals. Avoid sugar coated cereals or grains.

Choose fish, poultry or beans instead of red meats such as pork and beef. When you choose red meats, eat in small portions. When you eat out, choose foods that are low in calories, fats and sugar. Avoid large portions.

11.3 Watching Your Weight and Engaging in Physical Activity Help Prevent Cancer

There has recently been widespread concern about the epidemic proportions of obesity in the USA.

Obesity as a result of excesses in the diet and/or low physical activity increases the risk of cancer through a number of hormonal mechanisms in breast, endometrial and prostate cancer.

The increase in esophageal refluxes with obesity affects the appearance of Barrett's metaplasia (pre-malignant entity) and esophageal cancers. Esophageal adenocarcinoma, colon and rectal cancers, cancers of the kidney, pancreas, endometrium and breast have all been associated with excessive weight and obesity. These new facts keep us up to date in the fight against cancer through identifying groups with unhealthy habits and high cases of cancer that can be reduced by using life-saving strategies and interventions to improve lifestyle and support healthy environments.

In the United States, 2 out of every 3 adults are overweight or obese and less than half do sufficient physical activity.

Among children and young people, 1 out of every 3 is overweight or obese, and less than 1 of every 4 secondary school students fulfills the recommended levels of physical activity.

Obesity and physical inactivity are critical problems that every state is confronting. Among non-smokers, excess weight and a lack of adequate physical activity can be the most important risk factors related to cancer.

11.3.1 Recommendations for Weight Management

Ideally you should adopt an active lifestyle. For adults, at least 30 minutes of moderate physical activity (such as walking, dancing, gardening etc.) or strenuous physical activity (jogging, running, tennis etc.) is recommended for 5 or more days a week in addition to usual physical activity. Physical activity for 45 to 60 minutes is preferable. For children and adolescents at least 60 minutes of moderate or strenuous physical activity at least 5 days a week is recommended.

11.4 Sun Safety to Avoid Cancer

Epidemiological studies have shown the correlation between accumulated exposure to ultraviolet radiation (UV) and the risk of suffering from skin cancer.

A history of suffering from severe sun exposure while sunbathing, especially during infancy and adolescence, is associated with the risk of suffering from a melanoma in adulthood.

Evidence has shown that the UV rays from sunlamps or tanning lamps are carcinogenic. The use of artificial UV radiation increases the risk of suffering from skin cancer, especially basal cell carcinoma, squamous cell carcinoma and malignant melanoma particularly with the use of tanning lamps before the age of 35. Within this group of skin cancers, the melanoma is the most aggressive and fatal.

Approximately 30 million Americans visit tanning salons once a year. Women and young people are the most frequent users. The cosmetic tanning industry using UVA rays has responded to the risks of the use of artificial tanning by promoting campaigns that its' use is healthy. The tanning industry promotes campaigns such as "safe tanning" and its positive effects in the production of vitamin D. However, the most modern tanning lamps that emit mainly UV rays are inefficient for the synthesis of vitamin D.

The FDA has restricted the use of these artificial sun beds by people under the age than 18. However young people continue to be the ones who visit these cosmetic centers the most. Currently clients visiting these tanning centers are asked to sign a consent form. In this document the risks of this type of cosmetic treatment as well as the risk of damage to the eyes are explained.

11.4.1 Measures for Preventing Skin Cancer

- Avoid the sun between 10 am and 4 pm.
- Wear clothes that prevent exposure to solar rays.
- Apply protective sun creams with a SPF of at least 15 (sun protective factor). A sun cream with a SPF of 15 can absorb more than 92 percent of ultraviolet radiation.
- Avoid the application of artificial ultraviolet light using sunlamps or tanning lamps.

11.5 Work and Environmental Factors for Preventing Cancer

For many centuries it has been known that certain occupations increase the risk of suffering from cancer. In the 18th century Dr. Percival Pott, an English surgeon, was the first to demonstrate the relationship between cancer and an occupational carcinogen.

Dr. Pott demonstrated that chimney sweeps were more likely to suffer from squamous cancer of the scrotum than the rest of the population due to their contact with the soot. One of the most recent and important occupational carcinogens recognized as such is asbestos, which is more prominent among construction workers, plumbers and shipyard workers. Asbestos has been strongly linked to the incidence of mesothelioma, lung cancer and possibly malignant diseases of the digestive tract. Other types of occupational carcinogens include inhalation of radon which occurs among uranium miners, and increases the risk of lung cancer. Various other organic and aromatic chemicals are linked to the risk of suffering leukemia and cancers of the urinary tract.

11.6 Prevention of Cancer Induced by Infectious Diseases

Human papillomavirus (HPV) infections are directly implicated in the etiology of cervical carcinoma, so measures aimed at preventing it are effective in the prevention of this tumor. Contraceptive barrier methods reduce the risk of cervical neoplasia by reducing exposure to HPV. HPV was discovered in 1907, but was not linked to cervical cancer until 1976. The vaccine for preventing the HPV infection was approved in 2000. The hepatitis B virus was discovered in 1967 and was linked to liver cancer in 1974. In 1984 it was demonstrated that both hepatitis B and liver cancer could be prevented by vaccination against hepatitis B. From then on, in certain countries around the world, the vaccination of newborns against the hepatitis B virus became a routine.

It is estimated that 20% of all cancers are caused by viruses. The development of this field of medical study is promising.

11.7 Important Advice to Help Avoid or Reduce the Risk Factors of Cancer

- Avoiding tobacco

- Maintaining a healthy weight

- Keeping mobile with regular physical activity

- Eating healthily with plenty of fruits and vegetables.

- Limiting alcohol consumption

- Protecting the skin

- Knowing the family history of cancer

- Doing regular cancer detection checks and tests (screening)

12 Chemoprevention

The use of chemical substances, of natural or artificial origin, to prevent the development of a cancer is based in the ability of some molecules to block the initiation phases or to compete with stimulating substances of proliferation of neoplastic cells. Although it is an attractive route, and methodologically solid for contributing to the reduction of the problem of cancer, the proof of its beneficial effect in the general population is complex, as large scale studies are required over a long period, especially considering that the laboratory findings are not always reproducible in human studies. However, nowadays we know that antiestrogens (tamoxifen and raloxifene) can prevent breast cancer, finasteride can prevent prostate cancer and aspirin can prevent colon cancer. Retinoids can inhibit laryngeal cancer and selenium is being tested for the prevention of prostate cancer. Despite this valuable information obtained in large scale clinical studies, this type of chemoprevention has not had much reception due to a large exposure of potentially toxic medications in normal people.

Within these substances, vitamin supplements have been proposed for the chemoprevention of a large number of tumors. For the US Preventive Services Task Force (USPSTF) there is insufficient evidence that vitamin supplements (vitamins A, C or E) reduce the risk of cancer, as many studies have not been adequately designed and in others the results have been contradictory. Currently, it is not possible to decide what the balance is between the benefits and potential inconveniences of routine vitamin A, C and E supplement use, multivitamin complexes or folic acid, or combinations of antioxidants.

More recent results show that beta-carotenes are associated with a reduction in the risk of colon cancer in patients who have never smoked or consumed alcohol, while they confer an increase in this risk among smokers or those whose consume alcohol.

12.1 Chemoprevention for Breast Cancer

While chemoprevention studies with retinoids have been carried out, the studies with tamoxifen have represented a great advance in this pathology. Various studies show the effectiveness of tamoxifen in the reduction of breast cancer incidences, both invasive and in situ. The NSABP study found a decrease of 50% of the recidivisms and of the appearance of contra lateral cancer in patients with invasive carcinoma. This beneficial effect, however, is associated with an increase in the appearance of endometrial cancer and thromboembolic phenomena (deep vein thrombosis, pulmonary embolism and cerebrovascular accidents).

For this reason the USPSTF dismisses its use for the general population, but recommends its value in common practice for doctors with their high risk patients. There is evidence that raloxifene also prevents the appearance of breast cancer in women at high risk, although like tamoxifen, it is associated with a greater risk of thromboembolic phenomena and has secondary symptomatic effects ("hot flushes"), although these have not been associated with an increase in the risk of suffering from endometrial cancer. In conclusion, the balance between benefits and therapeutic damage can be favorable for some women at a high risk, for which reason they should consider the possibility of suffering from unwanted side effects as well as individual preferences.

12.2 Chemoprevention for Prostate Cancer

Based on the knowledge of the processes that control its appearance, the possibility of reducing or preventing the appearance of cancer is tremendously high in this tumor by blocking of the andrological stimuli on the epithelium of the prostate. The PCPT study (Prostate Cancer Prevention Trial) is a study with a large scale aleatoric allocation, which aims to define the role that a 5-alpha-reductase inhibitor, finasteride, has in the prevention of this tumor in blocking the developing effect of dihydrotestosterone. Also vitamin E (alfa tocoferol, an inhibitor of the proliferation and synthesis of DNA) showed positive results in the prevention of prostate cancer in the Alfa Tocoferol-Beta Carotene Cancer Prevention Study (ATBC). Other studies undertaken demonstrated that vitamin E has a protective effect against prostate cancer in smoking and non-smoking patients.

Patients with cancer consistently have lower selenium serum levels than those in healthy control groups. In fact, in the study carried out by Clark for skin cancer, a reduction in the risk of suffering from prostate cancer by two thirds was accidentally discovered among patients treated with selenium supplements. After this study there were others that showed the protective effect of selenium. However, a group of doctors from the M.D. Anderson Hospital carried out a multicentric aleatoric study with a duration exceeding 5 years. This study showed that it had no protective effect against various types of cancer. The SELECT study, which is the largest study to have been conducted on prevention to date, has been launched and will last for 12 years. This study is designed to directly observe the effects of selenium and vitamin E, both combined and separate, in order to prevent prostate cancer.

12.3 Chemoprevention for Colon Cancer

The non-steroidal anti-inflammatories (AINES, NSAID), including piroxicam, sulindac and aspirin, prevent the appearance of adenomas and induce the regression of adenomas already present in individuals with colon cancer or familial polyposis. The clinical usefulness of these drugs stems from their ability to inhibit the activity of cyclooxygenase (COX), which is able to transform arachidonic acid to prostaglandins. The isoenzyme COX-2 is an important mediator for the responses under stress and is a mediator for pain and inflammation. Non-selective inhibitors of COX are Indocin, Clinoril and Feldene, among others. On the other hand, celecoxib is among the selective inhibitors of COX-2.

Aspirin and its relation to the prevention of colon cancer have been studied. Previous studies have suggested that aspirin can protect against colon cancer and others. The results of a multinational clinical study on the preventive effects of aspirin were recently presented and included 861 people with a recognized genetic predisposition to colon cancer who were followed for a maximum of 10 years. The participants had Lynch syndrome, a condition that represents around three to five percent of colon cancer cases. Approximately one in every 1,000 people has the syndrome. The results of the study indicate that taking aspirin can prevent colon cancer in people with a family history of the disease.

Celecobix has been approved by the FDA to prevent precancerous lesions in people with a genetic predisposition to suffer from colon cancer. The use of aspirin and other COX inhibitors is intended for those with Lynch syndrome and not for the general population. The true balance of benefits and risks is yet to be determined for these medications taken over long periods of time. We must not forget that aspirin and COX inhibitors cause gastritis and this can be dangerous when it turns into a hemorrhagic gastritis.

Taking aspirin or COX inhibitors should not take precedence over other screening methods such as fecal occult blood, colonoscopy, etc.

12.4 Chemoprevention for Lung Cancer

Vitamins A, E and beta-carotene were chosen by epidemiological studies and they have shown a correlation between high consumption of these and high serum levels of these micronutrients to a lower risk of cancer, especially lung cancer. These are antioxidant components that can impede the carcinogens from damaging the DNA and other cellular systems. However, studies such as the ATBC (Alpha-Tocopherol Beta Carotene), which included 29,133 chronic smokers or the CARET study (US Beta Carotene and Retinol Efficacy Trial), which included 18,314 American smokers over a duration of several years did not show any effect of the vitamins A, E and beta-carotene on the prevention of lung cancer or on the incidence rate and mortality of lung cancer.

13 Secondary Prevention

The goal of diagnosing in the pre-clinical detectable phase of cancer for its early treatment is the reduction of the prevalence of cancer. In other words, unlike primary prevention, this is not preventing the appearance of new cases, but rather advancing the diagnosis in order to detect cancer in the early stages with the idea that there is a greater likelihood it will be cured, therefore reducing the number of existing cases. Secondary prevention is based primarily on public education and screening programs for early diagnosis of cancer. These involve the use of tests that are easily applicable at a national level, considered valid, financially affordable and accepted by health professionals and the public they are directed towards.

13.1 Public Education Programs

Their function is to transmit the necessary knowledge to the public to enable them to recognize "alarm" symptoms or signs that should be evaluated by a medical professional. Early recognition of these symptoms and rapid professional response will make correct diagnosis and treatment in less developed stages of the disease possible, resulting in an increased survival rate and most likely a lower therapeutic morbidity.

13.1.1 Symptoms that May be Signs of Cancer

The most common symptoms in adults are changes in the habits of the bladder and intestines, throat pain that does not go away, unusual bleeding and bruising, swelling or tumors in the breast or another part of the body, indigestion or difficulty swallowing, obvious changes in a freckle and a persistent or hoarse cough.

Cancers in children, as in adults, are difficult to identify. Parents should make sure that their children undergo regular checkups and pay attention to uncommon symptoms or signs that persist. Questionable symptoms could include unusual masses or inflammations, pastiness and unexplained loss of energy, a sudden tendency toward bruising, limping or persistent localized pain, unexplained prolonged fever or illness, frequent headaches commonly accompanied by vomiting, sudden changes in sight, rapid and excessive weight loss.

13.2 Early-Diagnosis Programs

The aspects relevant to defining the early diagnosis programs include the characteristics of the disease, the characteristics of the diagnostic tests which are aimed at screening the population and the characteristics of the group that will be included in this. The diagnostic test, finally, must be highly sensitive, and so specific that it guarantees a high predictive value for a positive result. It also must be reproducible, simple in its application and, in addition to being comfortable; it must also be safe for the patient. The financial cost must be affordable, both for individuals in privately financed health care systems and for those in public health care systems, both of which include thousands of citizens. Let's examine the following screening programs which have yielded beneficial results in the cancer mortality rate.

13.2.1 Early-Diagnosis Program for Cervical Cancer

This is the most widely used early detection program in the world. Cervical cancer has a high prevalence with a long subclinical duration (3-10 years) and curative treatment in early stages of the disease. Vaginal cytology, which is simple, cheap, comfortable and sensitive, is used for the screening of this cancer.

The program is easily carried out, due to its low costs and the high adherence of the population at risk. A significant reduction in the incidence of invasive cancer (by 3-10 times) and in mortality for this disease has been shown among women who undergo screening tests. The more intense the monitoring is, the greater the reduction. Changes in the sexual habits of the population, as well as the recognition of the role of HPV in the genesis of this cancer, have modified our concept of it, which is recognized epidemiologically as a sexually transmitted disease. The molecular identification test for HPV is not recommended for screening, but is recommended in cases where the cytology is abnormal.

An early screening start is advocated, at 18 and no later than 21, and, in any case, once the person has engaged in sexual activity. It should be carried out annually, although women over 30 years old who have had at least 3 negative results can reduce the frequency to every 3 years. Women with prenatal exposure to dietilestilbestrol (DES) or with an HIV infection, weakened immune system due to organ transplants, chemotherapy or chronic treatment with corticosteroids should have shorter intervals due to their increased risk of suffering from the disease. As regards the upper limit, normally women over 65 years old with previous negative controls are excluded, or at 70 if they have 3 or more negative cytologies and after at least 10 years of normal cytologies according to the ACS (American Cancer Society).

Screening is not intended for women who have had a hysterectomy due to non-tumor pathology, although the recommendations described apply to women who have had a hysterectomy without the cervix being removal.

The examination for uterine cancer (Papanicolau test) should start at 21 years of age. Women between 21 and 29 should have this test every 3 years. There is now also a test called the HPV test. The HPV test should not be used in this age range unless it is needed after an abnormal result in the Papanicolau test.

Women between the ages of 30 and 65 should have a Papanicolau test and also a HPV test (called "co-testing") every 5 years. This is the preferred focus, but it is also OK to have a Papanicolau test every 3 years.

Women over 65 who have had regular tests for cervical cancer with normal results do not need to continue with the Papanicolau tests. Women who have been diagnosed with pre-malignant lesions of cervical cancer (moderate/severe dysplasia or cancer in situ or also called CIN III) or who have been cured of an incipient cancer of the cervix should continue with the Papanicolau tests for at least 20 years after the diagnosis, also the tests should continue beyond the age of 65.

Women who have had their uterus removed (and also the cervix), for reasons unrelated to cervical cancer and who do not have a family history of cervical cancer or serious pre-cancerous lesions do not require regular Papanicolau tests. Papanicolau tests are carried out by gynecologists or obstetricians. These professionals are very familiar with the procedure for this test, which does not affect the virginity of patients who are virgins.

13.2.2 Early-Diagnosis Program for Breast Cancer
This is the most common tumor for western women and its early diagnosis not only carries with it a greater chance of a cure, but also avoids performing a serious mutilation such as a mastectomy.

Some potential screening procedures, specifically monthly breast self-examination and breast examination by a professional, are new no longer recommended due to their inefficiency in the reduction of mortality and the associated inconveniences, specifically the higher frequency of false positives, unnecessary biopsies and patient anxiety.

The method of choice is the mammogram, able to detect up to 85 % of tumors in the pre-clinical phase, a percentage that justifies the importance of these programs for itself. Mammograms allow for the detection of tumors that cannot be identified in a clinic. There is, however, debate about who should be screened, the type of mammogram, the reading method and those for revision and diagnostic confirmation. Currently it is recommended to start at 40, carrying out a double mammography projection annually or every 2 years, without an upper age limit. In Swedish programs a total reduction in mortality of 30% has been achieved, which reached 40% in women over 50 years old, the age at which the risk of cancer is clearly significant, and at which intervention greatly affects survival. In contrast, between the ages of 40 and 50, the reduction does not seem to be greater than 10%. For this reason, and considering the resources and health care structure in each country, the starting age can acceptably be a little later.

The recommendations of the ACS for early diagnosis of breast cancer are:
• Annual mammograms from 40 onward, continuing through the period during which a woman is in a good state of health.
• Clinical breast examinations more or less every 3 years for women in their 20s and 30s and every year for women aged 40 and over.

- Self-examination of the breast after menstruation every 2-3 months by women from the age of 20 onward. Women should know how their breasts normally look and feel and immediately report any change in the breast to their healthcare provider.

For some women, due to their family history, genetic tendency or to other factors, the breasts should be examined with magnetic resonance, in addition to mammograms. The number of women who fall into this category is minimal, less than 2% of all women. If you have a family history of breast cancer, ovarian cancer or other types of cancers, speak with your doctor about your history and whether you should undergo additional tests at an early age.

13.2.3 Early-Diagnosis Program for Colon Cancer

The early diagnosis programs should form part of the routine medical examinations for people over the age of 50. Detection of the disease in its early stages not only increases the survival rate, but also reduces mutilations due to amputation of the colon and rectum due to extensive surgery in the abdomen.

The fecal occult blood test has been associated with reductions in mortality which oscillates between 15% and 33%, in accordance with various studies, accepting an average reduction of 25%.

Furthermore it increases the percentage of tumors that are diagnosed while they are still localized by between 6% and 33%. It is a cheap and simple test, although the results are positive in only 1 to 5% of the general population. Approximately 2 to 10% of those with a positive result will have cancer, and 20-30% will be adenomas. Due to this elevated frequency of false positive results, its use carries with it a high use of confirmatory tests, such as colonoscopy, which decreases its cost-benefit analysis. In any case, the American health agencies recommend it annually from the age of 50 onward.

There are other noninvasive tests such as fecal immunohistochemical tests and DNA studies of the feces that are alternatives to the fecal occult blood test, but their role in the screening of colon cancer has yet to be defined.

The rectal tract is useful only for rectal lesions situated at least 7 cm from the anal margin, and its sensitivity has diminished for this group of cancers due to the increase in the proximal location of colon cancer. Flexible sigmoidoscopy reaches up to the last 60 cm of the colon, and its use, associated with the fecal occult blood test, has been proven to reduce mortality. With at risk patients, it is necessary to complete the study with an examination of the whole colon using colonoscopy.

For a study of the whole colon, it is also possible to use a tomography with a contrast agent, but its performance is no better than that of colonoscopy. Colonoscopy, in addition to having greater sensitivity and specificity, has the advantage of allowing a histological study and the removal of polyps. The high probability of the appearance of various tumors along the whole colon, due to the linking of the carcinogens by the feces, justifies the complete study using this procedure in principle, but its discomfort and possible complications can certainly limit its usefulness.

More recently so-called virtual colonoscopy, or colonography, has been introduced, which is a procedure in which the images of the colon constructed from the images obtained in the abdominal TAC are analyzed.
The expert consensus is that for the general population over 50 without risk factors, an annual fecal occult blood test should be carried out and the screening program below should be followed:

• Flexible sigmoidoscopy every 5 years or,
• Colonoscopy every 10 years or,
• Double contrast barium enema every 5 years or,
• Colonography by computerized tomography (virtual colonoscopy) every 5 years

In the high risk group (familiar poliposis adenomatosa, families with Lynch Syndrome, family history of colon cancer or polyps, ulcerative colitis, personal history of cancer or polyps), the screening recommendations logically shorten the periods and speed up the start, varying according to the choice of the patient and their doctor.

13.2.4 Early-Diagnosis Program for Prostate Cancer

Early diagnosis of prostate cancer is controversial, not only due to the lack of clear advantages in terms of survival, but also to the advanced age of the patients diagnosed, the different treatment options and their consequences. Effectively, while prostate cancer is a common disease, with a long pre-clinical stage, for which there are adequate treatments and simple, comfortable and affordable diagnostic tests, such as the rectal tract and determination of PSA (prostate-specific antigen that arises in prostate cancer) in the blood, consistent results in terms of survival have not been observed.

Screening for prostate cancer can carry with it false positive results, unnecessary biopsies and, above all, treatment of tumors that may never have affected the survival of the patient. However, the ACS recommends this program for patients older than 50 with the hope of living more than 10 years longer, starting at age 45 in men at high risk (blacks and people with a first-degree family history), and always notifying the uncertainties regarding the benefits and risks.

According to ACS, screening should, be carried out in those men who ask for it, whatever the case, considering it inappropriate not to offer the test or to advise against it.

It is appropriate however for men from the age of 50 onward speak with their doctor about the pros and cons of screening tests (PSA or rectal tract) so that they can decide if the test is the correct choice for them. Men who are black or have a father or brother who had prostate cancer before 65, should speak with a doctor about this from the age of 45.

13.2.5 Early-Diagnosis Program for Endometrial Cancer

The American Cancer Society recommends that at the onset of menopause, women should be informed of the risks and symptoms of endometrial cancer. Women should inform their doctors of any unexpected bleeding or marking after the symptoms of menopause have disappeared. Women who have had breast cancer and who receive treatment with tamoxifen and raloxifene have a 2 to 3 times greater risk of suffering from endometrial cancer and uterine sarcoma than the rest of the population. These patients should be evaluated by the gynecologist from the start of their treatment and should follow a program of periodical gynecological checks accompanied by a study of the thickness of the uterus with a trans-vaginal sonography. A biopsy of the endometrium is recommended if any thickening of the walls of the uterus is noticed.

13.3 Other Screening Programs

Although lung cancer is a common disease, the attempts to develop early detection programs have not yielded results, not only because we do not have effective treatments, but also because the pre-clinical detectable phase for the disease is short. The programs have included the use of chest x-rays and sputum cytologies, without significant increases in the survival rate, even with people of high risk.

For the disease referred to as ovarian cancer, it is not just one disease for which reason we do not have adequate early diagnostic methods. The use of CA-125 and ultrasounds has been proposed, without having demonstrated significant advantages, that is why it continues to be diagnosed in its advanced stages, which is its common form of clinical presentation.

Gastric cancer has been a target of focus due to its high incidence of it in certain countries, particularly Japan. In these frequent conditions, endoscopy and gastrointestinal transit seem to increase survival. Lastly, for other tumors, such as bladder cancer, the existence of "warning signs" (bruising) allows for the diagnosis of the disease in its early stages, for which reason, not having simple and trustworthy tests has not been an objective of systematic public early diagnostic programs.

www.ingramcontent.com/pod-product-compliance
Lightning Source LLC
Chambersburg PA
CBHW051252170526
45165CB00004B/1683